Physical Fitness Guide

JUST FOR YOU

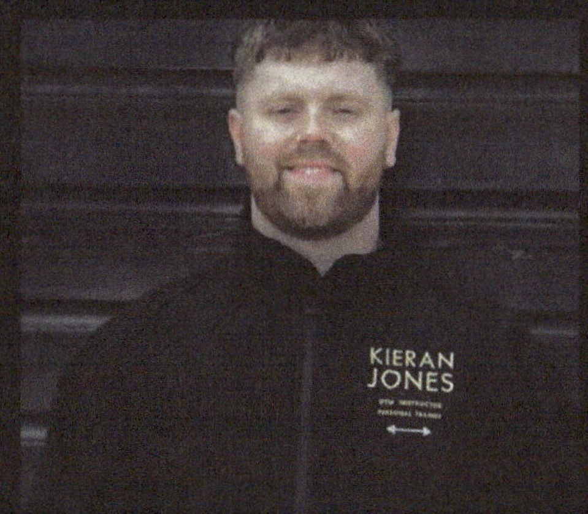

KIERAN JONES

GYM INSTRUCTOR | PERSONAL TRAINER

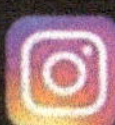 @kieranjonespt

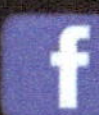 @kieranjonespt

AuthorHouse™ UK
1663 Liberty Drive
Bloomington, IN 47403 USA
www.authorhouse.co.uk
UK TFN: 0800 0148641 (Toll Free inside the UK)
UK Local: 02036 956322 (+44 20 3695 6322 from outside the UK)

This book is printed on acid-free paper.

ISBN: 979-8-8230-8439-0 (sc)
ISBN: 979-8-8230-8438-3 (e)

Library of Congress Control Number: 2023916592

Print information available on the last page.

Published by AuthorHouse 11/03/2023

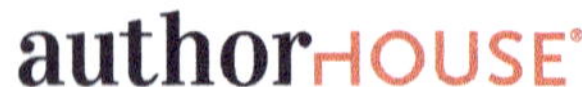

Physical Fitness Guide

JUST FOR YOU

Kieran Jones

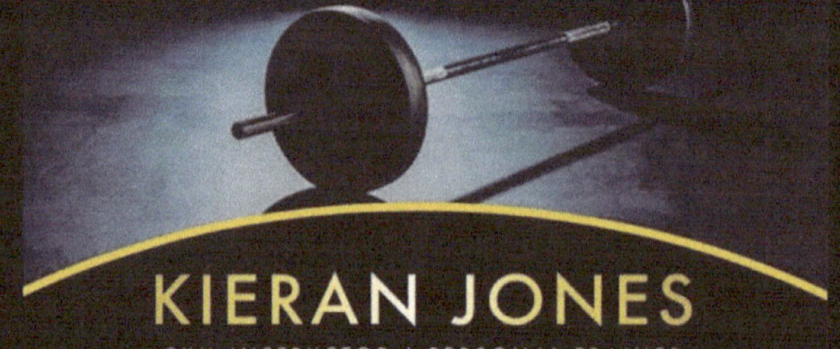

HIGH IN PROTEIN

- Eggs (white only)
- Fish (Tuna, Cod, Salmon, Herring)
- Greek Yoghurt
- Peanuts
- Cottage Cheese
- Chickpeas
- Almonds
- Peanut Butter
- Meat (Chicken, Turkey, Pork, Steak)
- Baked Beans
- Tofu
- Shrimps
- Prawns
- Broccoli
- Pumpkin Seeds
- Green Peas
- Chia Seeds
- Sausages

CARBOHYDRATES

- Apple
- Banana
- Quinoa
- Lentils
- Sweet Potatoes
- Potatoes
- Oats
- Rice
- Bread
- Kidney Beans
- Swede
- Strawberries
- Pears
- Grapes
- Oranges
- Crisps
- Cucumber
- Sugar
- Biscuits
- Carrots
- Courgette
- Pizza

HIGH IN FATS

- Cheese
- Butter
- Cashew Nuts
- Crisps
- Chocolate
- Avacado
- Olive Oil
- Salmon (omega 3 fats)
- Walnuts
- Full Fat Yoghurt

FIBRE FOODS

- Apples
- Raspberries
- Almonds
- Oats
- Brussel Sprouts
- Bran Flakes
- Muesli
- Sweet Potatoes
- Green Peas
- Kidney Beans
- Pears
- Whole Grain
- Kale
- Spinach
- Split Peas
- Baked Beans
- Almonds
- Coconut
- Pistachios

PROTEIN DRINKS

- Milk
- Huel
- Optimum Whey
- Optimum Mass Gainer
- BCCA's Drink/Tablet Form
- UFIT
- PHD Whey

ALCOHOL FATS

- Beer (154 cals)
- Ale (160-210 cals)
- Cider (249 cals)
- Lager (338 cals)

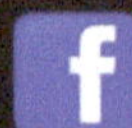 KIERANJONES FC/PT

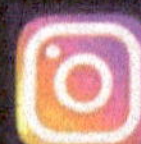 @KIERANJONESPT

KIERAN JONES

GYM INSTRUCTOR | PERSONAL TRAINER

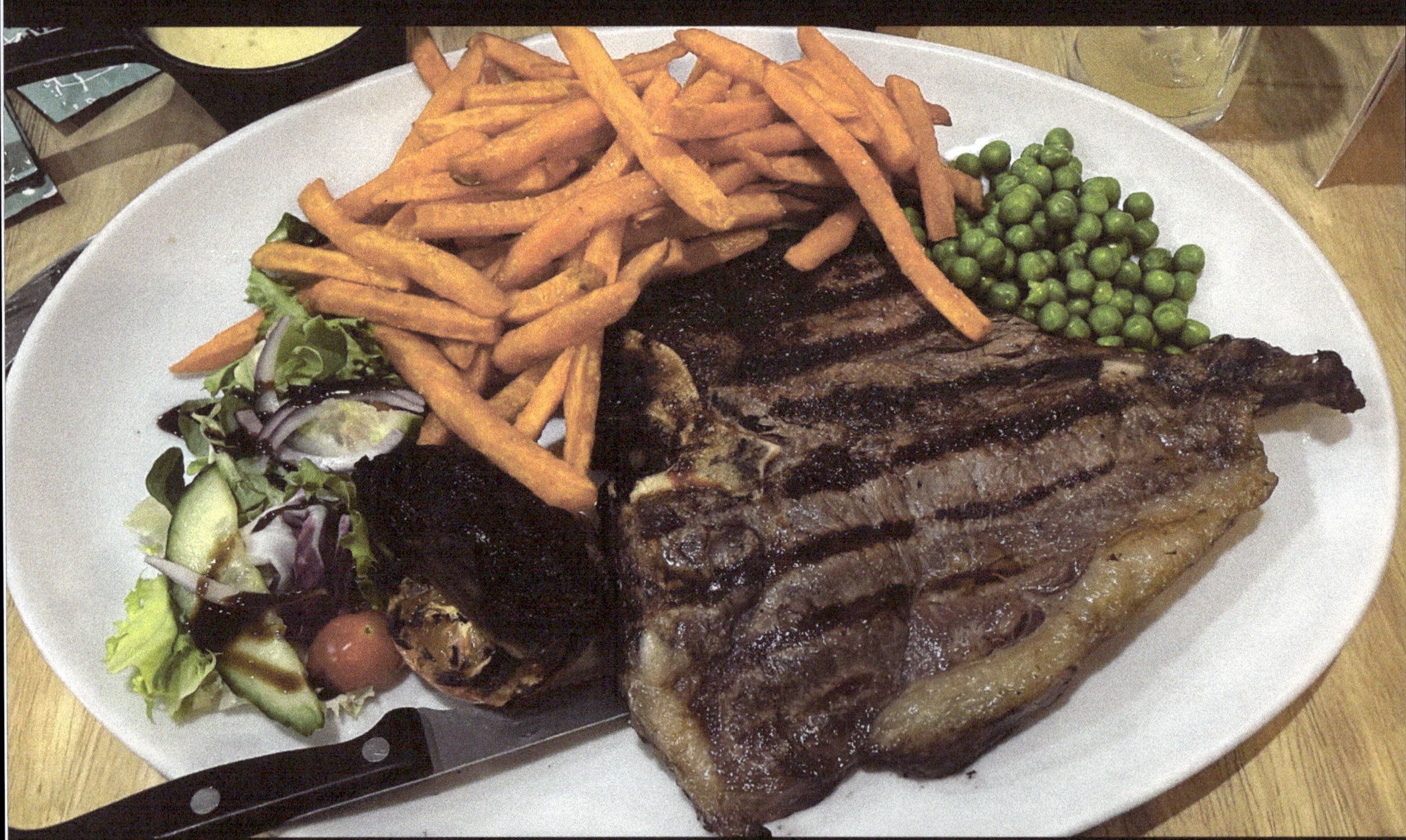

Macros

You may be reading this page and thinking to yourself, how I do track my calories?

Good question.

Using MyFitnessPal is the easiest and quickest way to track them.

We track them because it helps us as humans to not over indulge in food we consume and to not under consume. Being close to the calorie target is fine.

Hitting each macro group—protein, carbs, fats—is important because we can often consume too much of one and not enough of another.

Consuming too many carbs or fats has its knock-on effects, giving us more energy to do daily activities but not enough for repair and recovery (protein).

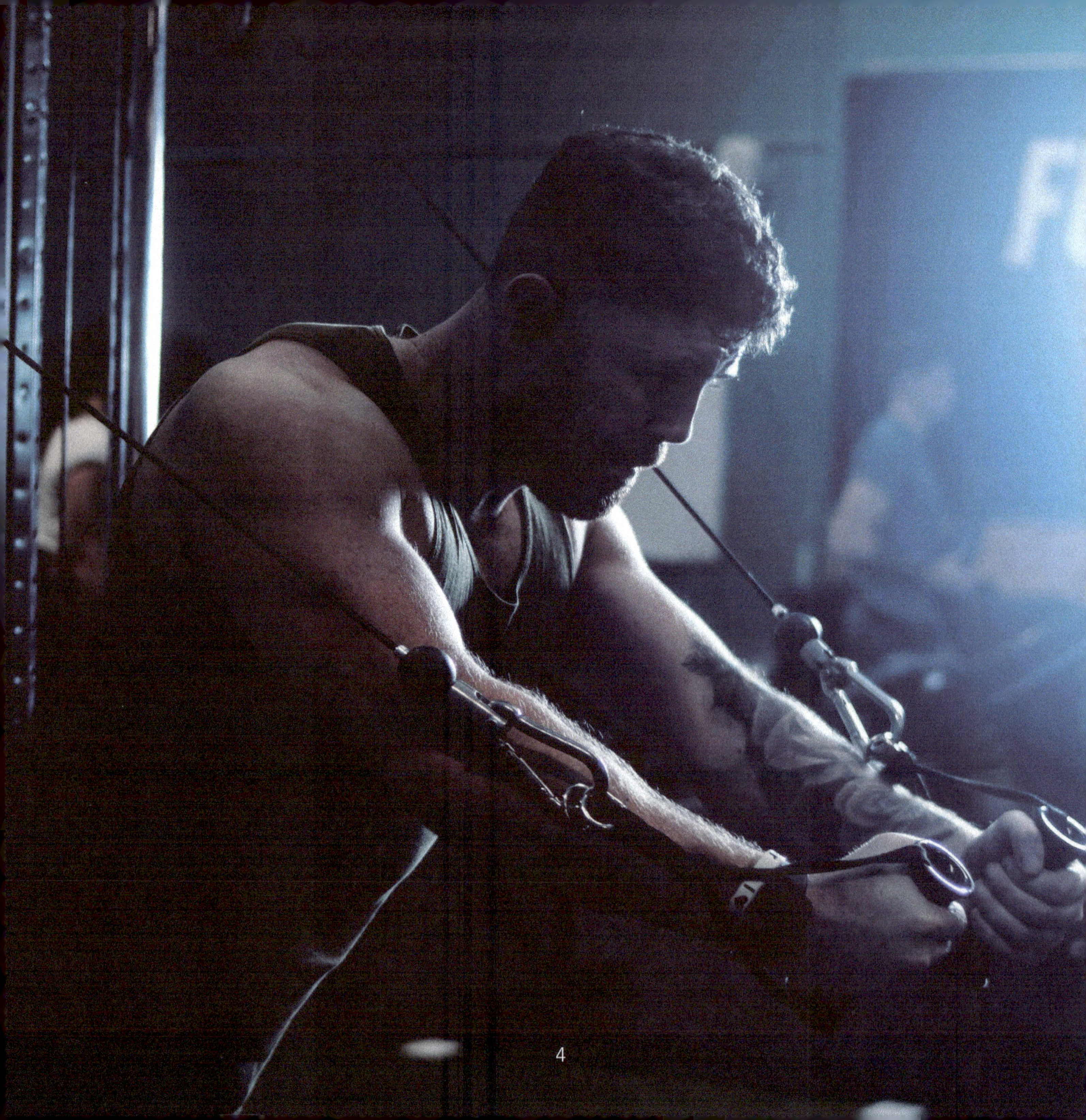

Benefits of Resistance Training

Resistance training is important to your workout regime due to the following benefits:

It burns a high amount of calories.

It is good for muscular endurance.

It improves muscle condition.

It improves flexibility and balance.

It offers chronic condition control.

It is good for aerobic activity.

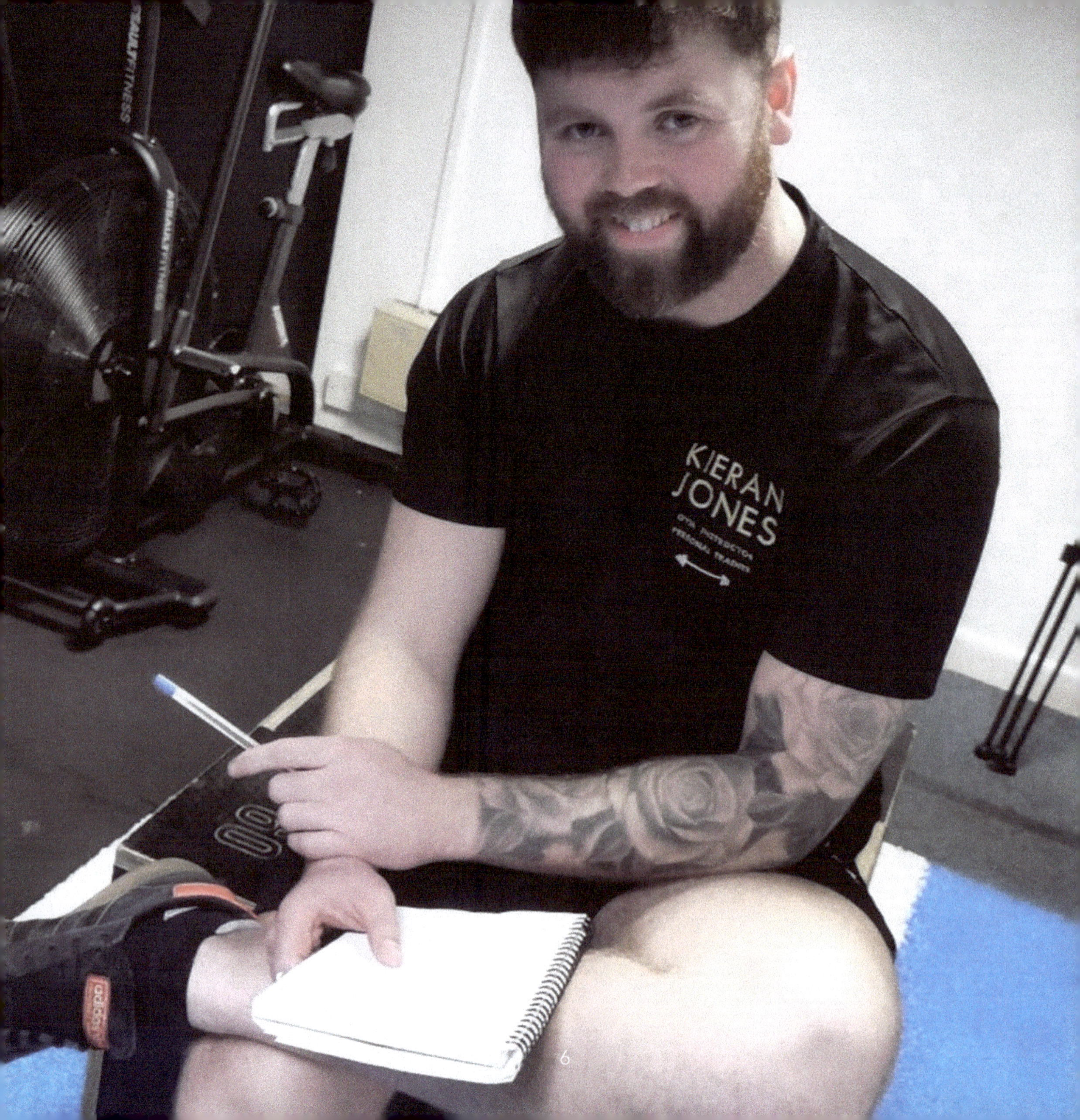
KIERAN
JONES
GYM INSTRUCTOR
PERSONAL TRAINER

Sticking to the Basics

Many of you overcomplicate exercise or even introduce new techniques to an exercise.

Sticking to the basics will help you learn step by step how to correctly perform your exercises.

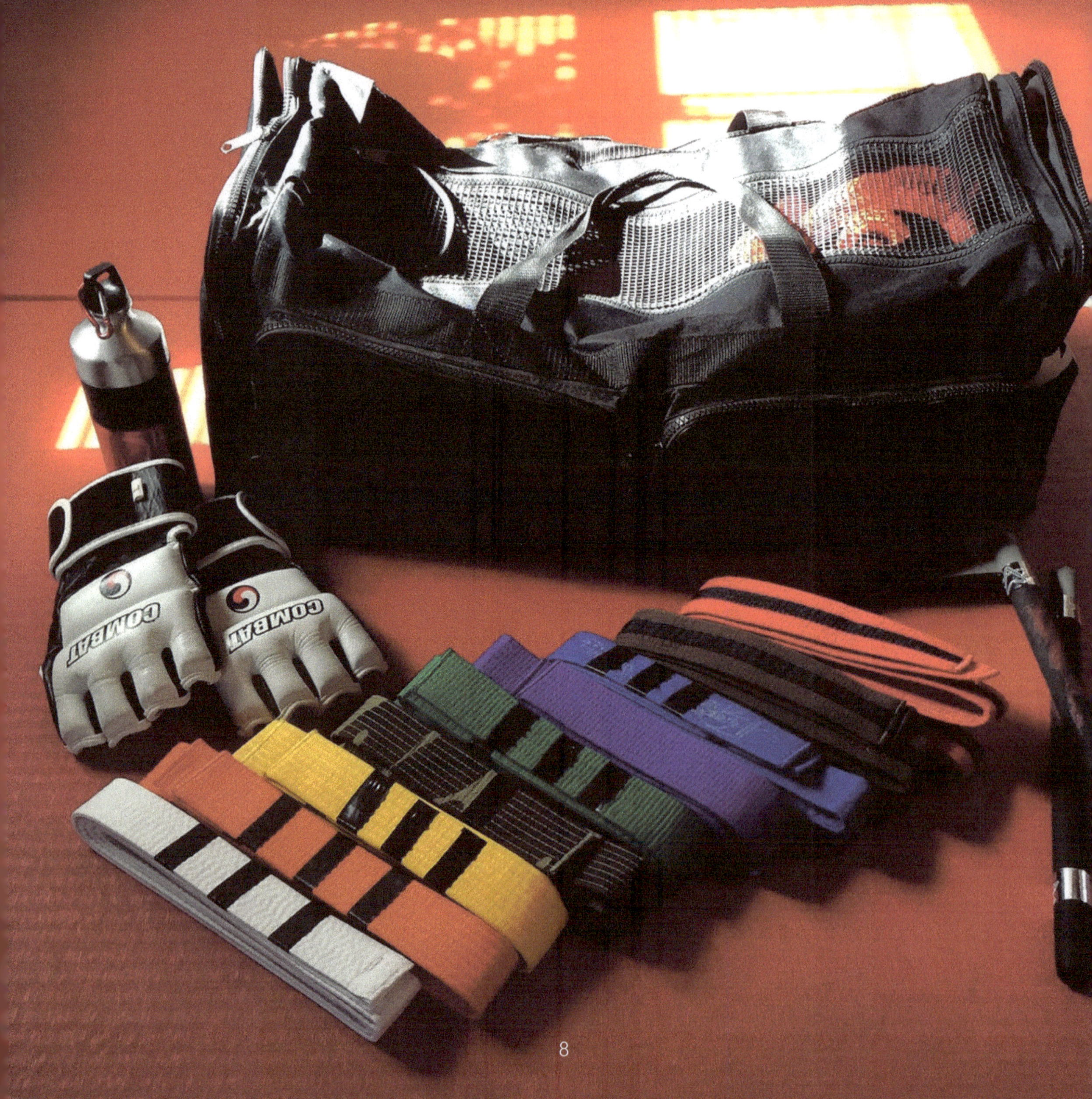

Gym Gear

Entering the gym with appropriate gym clothing is important. Some gyms will say you must wear certain clothes.

Wearing clothes that is comfortable for you—I'd say—*is* appropriate. Wearing vests or shorts or T-shirts that are either too tight or too small or even too big is uncomfortable.

Choose clothes you're happy with and that suit your body image. Being happy in your clothes when working out is beneficial for your self-esteem.

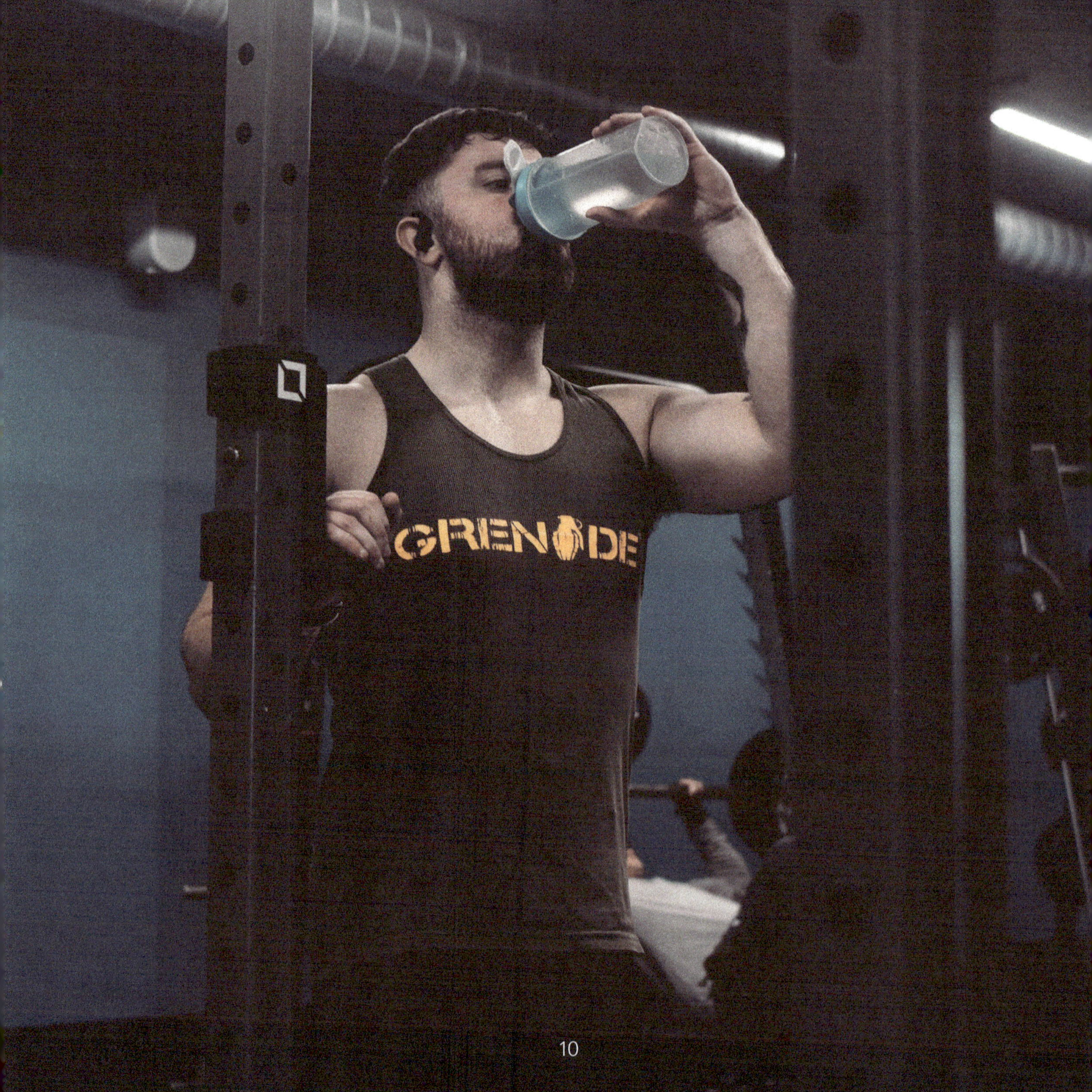

GRENADE

Keeping Hydrated

Keeping hydrated daily delivers benefits such as body temperature regulation and also keeps our organs functioning properly.

When water is consumed it enters the muscles and keeps the cells saturated. Cells also open for water to enter.

Water also helps with joint lubrication, which helps prevent injuries.

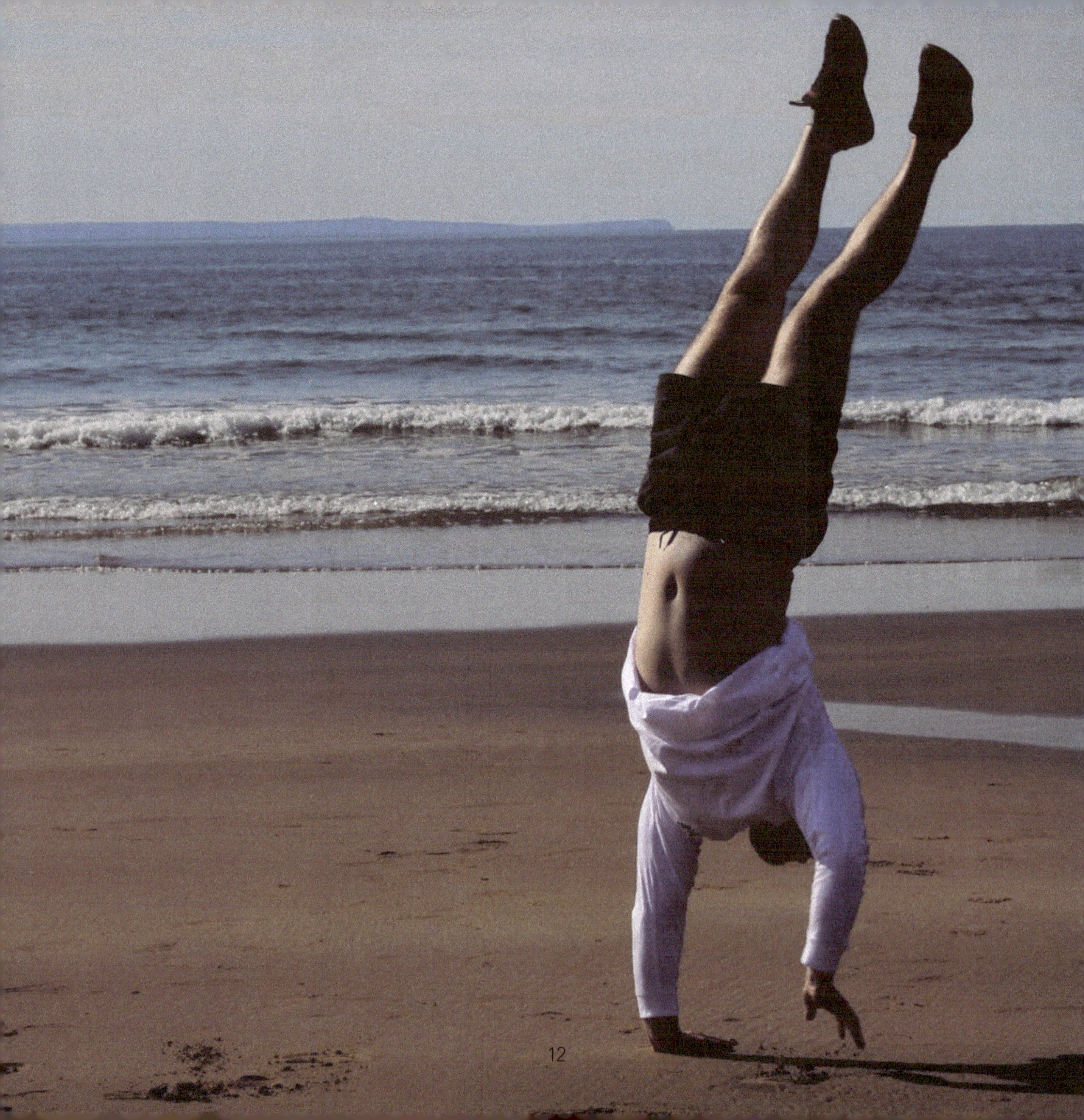

Rest and Recovery

We as human' need rest and recovery because when stressing the muscles they tear/rip, causing them to fatigue and making us tire quicker during our activities. A normal rest and recovery period is from between forty-eight and seventy-two hours.

Long rest and recovery times can also lead to less injuries.

NOTES

NOTES

NOTES

NOTES

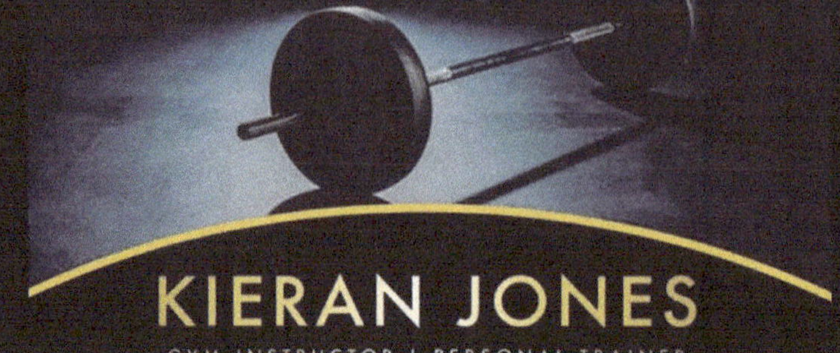

HIGH IN PROTEIN

- Eggs (white only)
- Fish (Tuna, Cod, Salmon, Herring)
- Greek Yoghurt
- Peanuts
- Cottage Cheese
- Chickpeas
- Almonds
- Peanut Butter
- Meat (Chicken, Turkey, Pork, Steak)
- Baked Beans
- Tofu
- Shrimps
- Prawns
- Broccoli
- Pumpkin Seeds
- Green Peas
- Chia Seeds
- Sausages

CARBOHYDRATES

- Apple
- Banana
- Quinoa
- Lentils
- Sweet Potatoes
- Potatoes
- Oats
- Rice
- Bread
- Kidney Beans
- Swede
- Strawberries
- Pears
- Grapes
- Oranges
- Crisps
- Cucumber
- Sugar
- Biscuits
- Carrots
- Courgette
- Pizza

HIGH IN FATS

- Cheese
- Butter
- Cashew Nuts
- Crisps
- Chocolate
- Avacado
- Olive Oil
- Salmon (omega 3 fats)
- Walnuts
- Full Fat Yoghurt

FIBRE FOODS

- Apples
- Raspberries
- Almonds
- Oats
- Brussel Sprouts
- Bran Flakes
- Muesli
- Sweet Potatoes
- Green Peas
- Kidney Beans
- Pears
- Whole Grain
- Kale
- Spinach
- Split Peas
- Baked Beans
- Almonds
- Coconut
- Pistachios

PROTEIN DRINKS

- Milk
- Huel
- Optimum Whey
- Optimum Mass Gainer
- BCCA's Drink/Tablet Form
- UFIT
- PHD Whey

ALCOHOL FATS

- Beer (154 cals)
- Ale (160-210 cals)
- Cider (249 cals)
- Lager (338 cals)

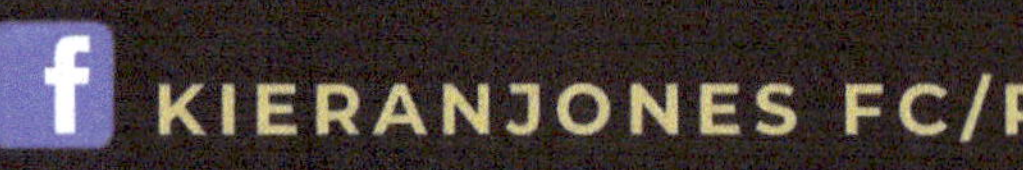

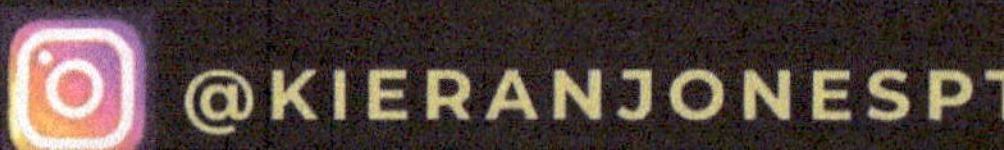

KIERAN JONES

GYM INSTRUCTOR | PERSONAL TRAINER

www.ingramcontent.com/pod-product-compliance
Lightning Source LLC
Chambersburg PA
CBHW040401240726
48664CB00012B/1703